SAVE TIME

with

Circuit Training

Lisa M. Wolfe

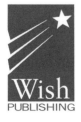

Wish Publishing
Terre Haute, Indiana
www.wishpublishing.com

LCCN: 2005927031

Editorial assitance provided by Dorothy Chambers
Cover designed by Phil Velikan
Cover photography and interior photography provided by Lisa M. Wolfe

Printed in the United States of America
10 9 8 7 6 5 4 3 2 1

Published in the United States by
Wish Publishing
P.O. Box 10337
Terre Haute, Indiana 47801, USA
www.wishpublishing.com

Distributed in the United States by
Cardinal Publishers Group
Indianapolis, Indiana 46264

For Nana,
who always encouraged me to follow my dreams

TABLE OF CONTENTS

1

Introduction to Circuit Training

ACE (The American Council on Exercise) predicted for the year 2004 a need for "faster, quicker workouts." Women living in the 21st century can certainly understand this need. Pressures from work, family and recreation fill up every minute of the day, leaving little personal time. Along with those pressures, the need to take care of ourselves exists. Taking care of our bodies without the sacrifice of two hours spent in the gym is the goal.

A circuit training workout fills that need for a faster workout that utilizes minimal equipment. For those of us who are time-starved, this workout provides a quick alternative to spending an hour exercising for cardiovascular health and fat burning, then an additional hour in the gym for strengthening.

If you've been doing the same exercises over and over for months at a time, it's time for a change! This workout can be performed inside or outside, during the day or at night, or in rainy weather. There is no dependence on weather, time or health club hours in order to get the workout that you need.

Circuit training is an exercise style, a type of interval training, which provides a total body workout in a quick amount of time. Another benefit is that it erases the boredom that often comes from indoor exercises, because the workouts are constantly changed. Every day the workout can be different, yet still provide the strengthening and overall body health benefits without spending two hours at a gym.

Circuit training is based on a set amount of time spent in different activities. It alternates bursts of intense activity with lesser intense activities. The workout consists of small stations, alternating a cardio-vascular exercise with a strengthening exercise. Once or twice through all the stations completes the circuit. The total time spent in each station can vary, but 1½ minutes in each works well. The workout can last anywhere from 20 to 60 minutes depending on the needs of the day. This workout should be performed with a day of rest in between to allow muscles recovery time.

More is not better with circuit training. Three to four days a week is sufficient to see changes in the body. The other days can be spent walking, bicycling, swimming, etc. When the workout is performed more frequently, the body spends energy and time recovering from the workout instead of delivering the strength gains.

Not only is circuit training an efficient workout style, it also helps to avoid injuries that come from repetitive activities and overuse. Since the exercise stations are changed every day, the body is allowed to work through the different planes and ranges of motion. This protects the joints and muscles as well as strengthens them in various positions. All together, that leads to injury prevention, avoidance and protection.

During the workout, different energy systems are used in the alternating stations. While one system is working, the other system is resting. This allows for a higher intensity work phase, increasing our benefits.

The workout can be used by anyone, at any age. For the older adult, circuit training is an "effective well-rounded exercise program that can be utilized as a means to improve health-related components of fitness in older adults," according to a study published in the *European Journal of Applied Physiology* in August 2004. The results of the study on 35 older adults indicated that circuit training elicits significant improvements in cardiorespiratory fitness, muscular strength, body composition and high-density lipoprotein cholesterol (the good one).

Along with being a fast, effective workout, circuit training challenges each body to its own personal limits. Those new to exercise can begin at a lower intensity and build at their own pace. Athletes can begin at a higher intensity and challenge their bodies in the areas where they want to see specific improvements. It is not a sport-specific style of training. Those training for sports need to apply certain adaptations in the stations. For example, a marathon runner would need to include more frequent running throughout the stations.

The workout uses the body's two energy systems: aerobic (meaning with oxygen) and anaerobic (meaning without oxygen). The aerobic system allows us to walk, run, bike, etc. for a long duration. The anaerobic system provides short bursts of energy in order to jump, lift heavy weights or sprint. Since oxygen is not used in this system, the muscles respond with a burning sensation, the buildup of lactic acid. That sensation indicates we are strengthening the muscles.

Circuit training maintains the heart rate at an increased level to allow for aerobic conditioning throughout the entire workout. Even during the strengthening exercises, the heart rate will not recover to the resting rate. This constant elevation requires the body to use fat as the energy source, leading to reduced weight levels and lower body fat percentages.

The strength gains through the workout increase muscle tissue in the body. The increased muscle tissue, in turn, increases the body's metabolism. Unlike body fat tissue, muscle tissue requires more calories to function in a day, so our body uses the food we eat as energy to maintain this lean body mass as opposed to storing the food intake as fat.

Another benefit of circuit training is it can be performed solely by using the body in various positions. There is no need for a lot of equipment or large exercise machines. It can be practiced anywhere, indoors or out. However, there are some recommendations for an indoor, at-home workout: use a stopwatch, timer or clock to keep track of the time in each station; locate a space in which to move around and not be compromised; dumbbells, benches, balls and mats should also be in the room with the exercise stations set up prior to beginning the workout.

It's also a good idea to write down the order of the stations so time will be spent exercising and not wondering what comes next. Included in the back of the book are cut-out pages with a sample workout for your convenience. Spend a few weeks rearranging the order of those exercises until you are comfortable adding your own personal favorites. When arranging the order of the strength stations begin with a large muscle group and work down to a smaller group. For example, begin with the legs or back and progress through the chest, abdominals, arms and finally shoulders or calves.

If treadmills, stationary bikes, medicine balls, resistance bands or more are available, those can be included in the stations. Get creative in the design of the stations. Change them to provide a different workout each time. Use what is available and even what your children have (trampolines, pogo sticks, etc.) to make it an entertaining and effective workout!

2

Body Overview

The body is a fascinating machine. Each body is made differently. That's how we tell each other apart. It's important not to put yourself in competition with anyone else. Your body is not going to look like anyone else's no matter how hard you try.

Real fitness is about accepting your body the way it is. We have to work within our own personal and genetic limitations to make this body the best it can be. It's the only one we get and it has to last 80 to100 years.

When it's operating at peak performance, the body makes us feel as if we can accomplish anything. To understand more, we can take a look at what's occurring underneath the skin.

Even a simple movement requires precision by the muscles, joints, nerves and bones. Through the spinal column runs our central nervous system which is the control center for the body. Messages are relayed from the brain through the central nervous system and out to the corresponding limbs, bones and muscles to produce the movement.

The cardiovascular system contains the heart, blood and blood vessels. This system works to aid in the flow of oxygen and nutrients to the cells, carries waste from the cells, helps to regulate body temperature and regulates blood flow to prevent serious blood loss.

Our respiratory system brings in oxygen we breathe for use in the blood, tissues and cells. The lungs aid in the gas exchange to the blood, bringing in oxygen and releasing carbon dioxide. Cardiovascular exercise helps to strengthen these systems and make them more efficient. The cardiorespiratory system working together is what allows us to maintain exercise for 30 to 40 minutes.

Our digestive system converts the food we eat into energy. A variety of foods is available to us to satisfy the needs of the body. The key to healthy eating is to eat a variety and to eat in moderation. Eat when you're hungry and eat until you're full. Have on hand healthy snacks, so you will not be tempted to snack on junk food.

If you think you're going to lose weight by not eating, you're wrong. When you don't eat, the body holds food like a squirrel storing his nuts in his cheek for the winter. Your body doesn't know when you're going to feed it again, so anything you put in gets stored as fat in order to prevent starvation. It is necessary to feed the body every few hours, so the food can be used as energy instead of stored as fat.

Breakfast is important. Did you know that sumo wrestlers skip breakfast in order to be hungrier later in the day? This allows them to eat larger meals later and pack the weight on. Not a good goal for us!

Skipping breakfast, according to obesity specialist Dr. Wayne Callaway at George Washington University, can not only trigger over-eating later in the day but can also cause a drop in metabolism. He found that people who skip breakfast have a 5-percent lower metabolism than those who don't skip breakfast. He explains that eating (digesting and absorbing the food) raises metabolism, so skipping meals can lower the metabolic rate slightly.

Our metabolism goes to sleep at night, just like we do. If we wake at 6 o'clock and do not eat until 11 o'clock, we've lost five hours of our metabolism working for us. We do not need a large breakfast. A bowl of cereal, piece of fruit, or eggs and toast will be enough to wake that metabolism up with us.

Our system also needs water. Seventy-five percent of our muscles are composed of water. It contains important nutrients to keep us operating at an efficient level. Lack of water makes us feel tired, confused and unmotivated. Thirst is not an adequate indication for water level. If you're thirsty, you're already on your way to dehydration. The average adult should drink eight glasses of water every day.

Think of your body like an empty milk jug. You wouldn't use juice, pop or more milk to clean out that jug. You would use water. It's the same for our bodies. We need to keep them clean from the inside out with continuous water flowing through.

The skeletal system is made up of 206 bones. The bones provide protection for the organs, support for soft tissue, which allows us to stand, and a basis on which muscles move. Bones also produce certain blood cells and store calcium, sodium and other minerals. Strength training helps to build the density of the skeletal system, preventing osteoporosis.

Osteoporosis is a weakening of the bones. The bones' porosity increases, making us more susceptible to injuries. Osteoporosis usually occurs as one ages. One reason for this is the fact that calcium can be stored in the bones only until the early thirties. From that point on, our job is to maintain our stores through eating calcium-rich foods such as milk, yogurt and cheese. We can also increase the density of the bones through strength training or weight-bearing exercises such as walking, dancing and jogging.

The core of our body provides stability and a base from which movement occurs. The core includes the spine and the muscles of the stomach and back. The spine is made up of 24 vertebrae (bones) that run from the neck through the tailbone. Muscles exist deep in the body next to the spine to support this structure. The body also has muscles that are closer to the surface in the back, chest and abdominal area. These muscles work together to maintain a strong trunk.

The abdominal muscles are a group of four different muscles. One runs up the center of the stomach. One runs around the stomach holding it in place and supporting posture. The other two cross over each other along the sides, similar to putting our hands in our front pockets and our back pockets. It is important to keep these muscles strong in order to prevent strain on the back.

The muscular system allows our body to move in many different directions. We can rotate, lift, bend, elevate and extend because of the pattern of the muscles in the body.

The lower extremity muscles allow our legs to kick, lift, ride a bike, point our toes, extend the knee, etc. These muscles activate the ankle, knee and hip joints. Keeping all the groups strong and working together helps to prevent joint pain and maintains proper range of motion.

The upper extremity muscles allow us to drive a car, write a letter, wave hello, wash our hair, etc. These muscles activate the shoulder, elbow and wrist joints. Keeping these groups strong aids in proper posture and improved self-confidence by confirming we can lift groceries, move furniture or carry our own luggage.

When beginning an exercise program to strengthen the muscles, follow a program that allows for individual variations and special considerations. Chapter 7 will address these concerns.

3

Cardiovascular Exercises

CARDIOVASCULAR

We've already talked a little about cardiovascular (CV) health and fitness. The CV system includes the heart, lungs, blood and blood vessels. To strengthen this system, cardio exercises such as walking, jogging, running, swimming, cycling or rollerblading need to be performed. These are exercises that elevate the heart rate for a specific amount of time and are aerobic exercises, or exercises that use oxygen.

Other benefits of CV exercise include lowered blood pressure, reduced feelings of stress, decreased body fat, increase in good cholesterol, decrease in bad cholesterol, loss of weight, decreased symptoms of depression, and reduced anxiety levels.

In order to be effective, CV exercise needs to be performed within a certain heart rate range. When the heart is working too hard, sugar is the energy, or fuel source. Sugar does not last long. It is the source used for quick bursts of energy such as sprinting. When the heart is not working hard enough, some CV benefits are occurring, but not a lot of weight reduction will be made.

When the heart is working in the correct range, fat is the energy, or fuel source. Fat is our endurance energy and will last for the 30 to 40 minutes that we need, such as in cross country running.

A simple indicator to measure the correct training range is the talk test. While exercising, you should be able to talk — carry on a conversation. If you're able to talk, you are working in the fat-burning range. If you're unable to talk, you're working too hard and burning sugar for energy. If you can sing, you're not working hard enough.

To more accurately measure the target heart rate range, we use the following formula:

220 - age x .6 = low range
220 - age x .8 = high range

For example, the heart rate range for a 30 year old would be 114 to 152 beats per minute (BPM).

220 - 30 = 190 x .6 = 114
220 - 30 = 190 x .8 = 152

If the heart rate falls below 60%, the body receives cardiovascular benefits, but not fat burning. If the heart rate increases too much over 80% the body burns sugar as the energy source instead of fat. Between 60 and 80%, the body improves cardiovascular health and burns fat as the fuel.

Calculate your heart rate range before a workout. Write it down and keep it accessible. While exercising, find the pulse either on the wrist or the neck. The heart rate can be found on the little-finger side of the back of the wrist, or on the side of the neck. Use the two fingers of your hand to feel for the pulse, not your thumb. The thumb has a pulse of its own. Count the number of beats in 10 seconds, and then multiply that answer by six. Your result should fall within your range.

To see benefits from cardiovascular training, the workout should be performed three to four days per week. The heart, lungs and fat cannot see which exercises you are doing, so it is important to choose ones that you enjoy. It also helps to vary the exercises to alleviate boredom.

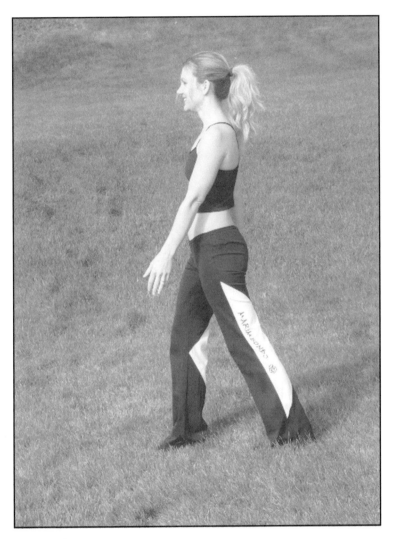

Walking

Walk around the room, landing on the heel and rolling through the toe. Take normal strides. Move the arms in an exaggerated movement to increase the heart rate. Vary this exercise by walking backward or sideways.

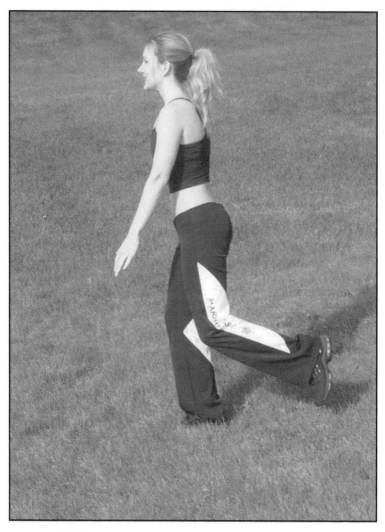

Jogging

Jog around the room. Jogging in place is not recommended since it causes strain on the knees. The movement can be forward, backward or sideways. Allow the arms to move as you're jogging. Remember to look straight ahead, hold your stomach in tight and keep your back straight with the body tall. You can also jog to the beat of fast music to increase the pace.

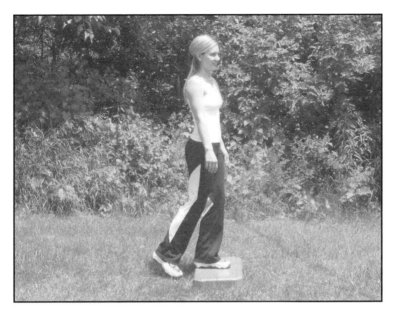

Step-ups

Step up and down, on and off of a bench. Begin with your right foot followed by the left for half of your station time. Then switch to the left foot first followed by the right for the remainder. Step down to the same side of the bench that you started from. It is not recommended that you step off the front side of the bench on the way down. You may also climb and descend stairs.

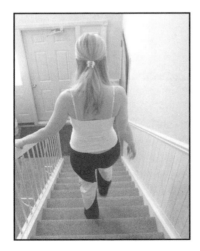
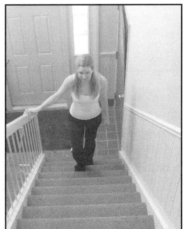

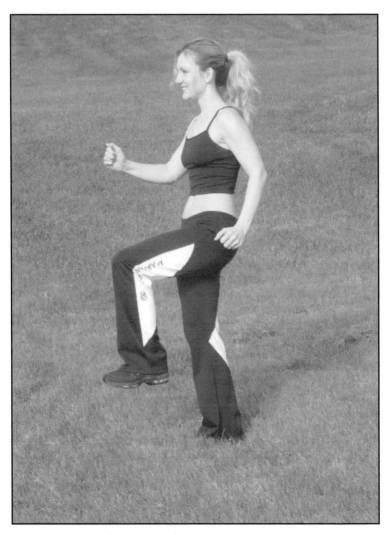

Marching in Place

Quickly march to the beat of the music. Bend your elbows at a 90-degree angle and pump the arms up and down in time with the feet. Raise the knees to a comfortable height in front of the body. Bring your full foot into contact with the floor, not just the toes.

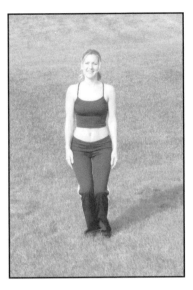
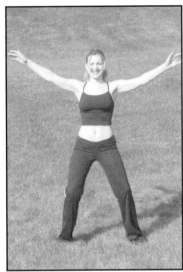

Jumping Jacks

Begin standing tall with feet together and arms at the sides. Jump and spread the feet apart as your arms extend overhead. When you land the feet keep a slight bend in the knees. Quickly jump and bring your feet back together and return arms to the sides. Repeat the movement without a rest in between.

Time Saving Tips

- Three 10-minute sessions of exercise a day provide the same benefits as one 30-minute workout.
- Use the stairs instead of elevators and park farther away from stores to add bits of exercise to your day.
- Plan ahead for your workout. Keep your exercise equipment easily accessible.
- Schedule exercise into your day.
- Have a purpose to your workout.
- A year from now you may wish you had started exercising today.

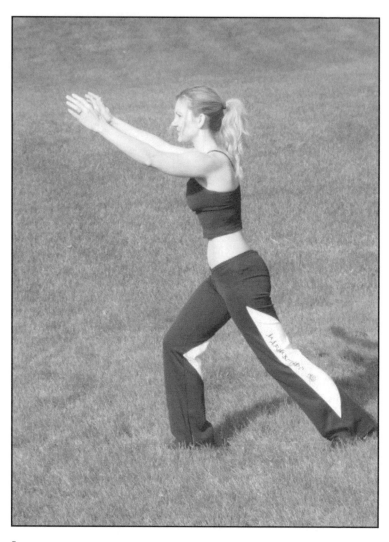

Lunges

Quickly alternate lunge steps behind the body. Swing the arms out in front of the body when the foot steps back. Do not bend the front knee more than 90 degrees and keep the front knee in line with the front heel. Do not bring the knee forward over the toes. On the step back, tap the foot to the floor and then return it alongside your other foot.

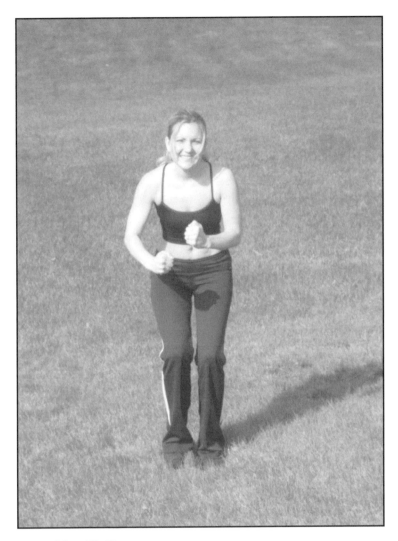

Football Run

Rapidly run in place. Keep your feet close together and close to the ground. Bring your hands into fists in front of the body. Pump the hands up and down in an exaggerated movement while running. For a variation, you can run forward, backward, side to side or around in small circles.

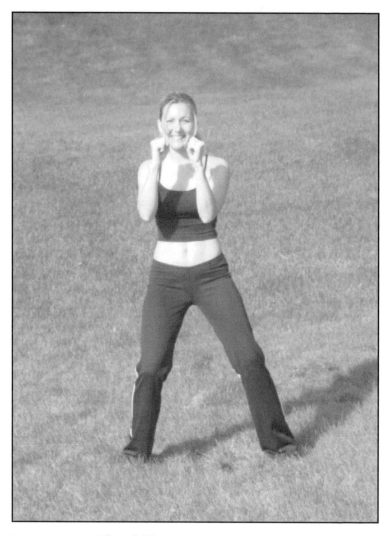

Boxer's Shuffle

Begin standing with your feet slightly wider than hip distance apart. Keep your knees and toes facing the same direction. Keeping the knees slightly bent, move the feet in a fast shuffle to the right and back to the left. Place the hands in fists next to your face.

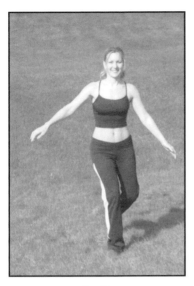 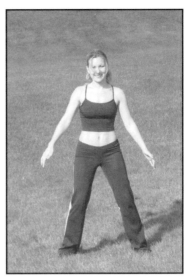

Hopscotch

This exercise is performed just like the children's game. Move forward by first hopping on one foot, then two, one foot, then two. For equal benefit to both legs, alternate right and left feet when landing on the single foot.

CV Exercise Can Be a Family Activity Too

- Follow the leader is an excellent example of a circuit workout. The leader runs, walks, jumps, rolls, squats, plays hopscotch and the rest follow along behind.
- Children enjoy exercise too. You can set up a mini-circuit on those stay-indoors days. Put on some silly music and lead the children through a workout with stations they'll enjoy.
- Some of the best family memories are made while doing a physical activity. A nature walk, beach swim, tree climb or a game of basketball are all moments to talk while improving your health.

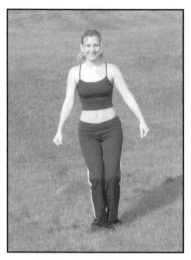
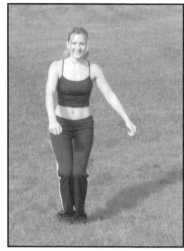

Downhill Ski Jumps

Begin standing with feet and knees together. Bend your knees slightly and jump feet to the side, as if jumping over an imaginary line. Land and quickly jump back over the line. Use the arms side to side to add to the propulsion. Think of simulating downhill mogul skiing.

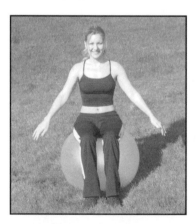
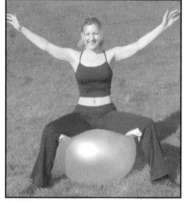

Jumping Jacks on Ball

Sit on the ball with legs close together and arms at the sides. Begin bouncing up and down. On a bounce, widen your legs and arms out to the sides. On the next bounce, close legs and arms. Sit tall with your back straight and your stomach held in tight.

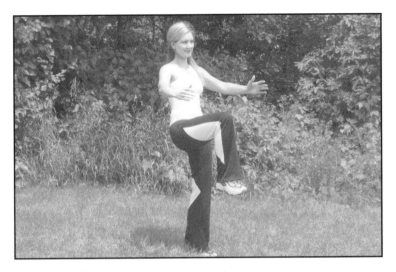

Knee Lifts

Stand tall with arms overhead. Lift your right knee up to the level of the hips as the arms pull down. Set the right foot down and return arms overhead. Lift your left knee up to the level of the hips, pulling the arms down. Set the left foot down. Continue changing sides and lifting the knees as quickly as possible.

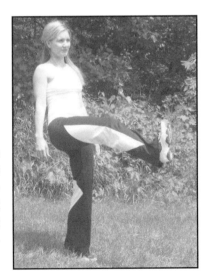

Front Kicks

Stand tall and leave the arms at the sides. Lift your right knee and then extend the leg out kicking with the heel. Bend your right leg and then set the right foot down. Repeat with the left. Continue alternating the kicks.

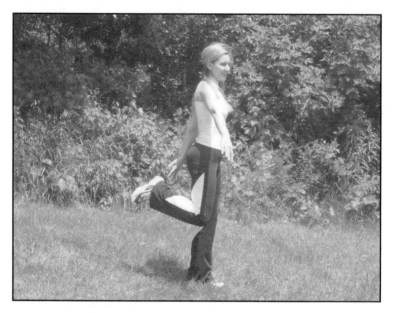

Heel Touches

Stand tall with arms at the sides. Bend the right knee underneath the body, bringing your right foot toward your behind. Reach your left hand behind the body toward the right foot. Alternate these heel touches quickly, with or without a hop in between.

Think FITT!

Frequency: 3-6 days a week
Intensity: your heart rate range
Type: use exercises that you enjoy
Time: 30-60 minutes

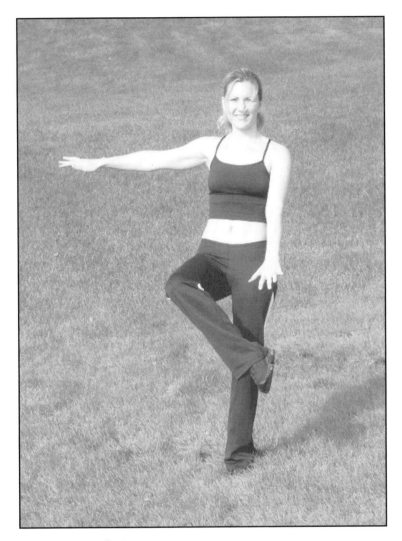

Soccer Kicks

Begin standing tall with arms out to the sides at shoulder level. Bend your right knee toward the outside of your body. This will bring your heel toward the front of your body, as if kicking a soccer ball. Reach down with the left hand toward the right heel. Quickly alternate these soccer kicks with or without a hop in between.

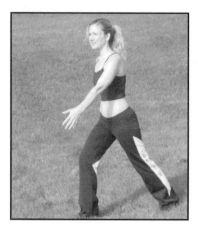
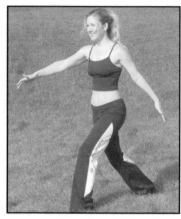

Cross Country Ski

Stand tall with your right foot approximately two feet in front of your left foot. Stretch your left arm out in front of the body. Jump and switch your right and left feet. Land with your left leg in front and right arm stretched out.

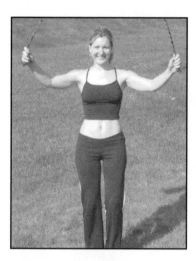
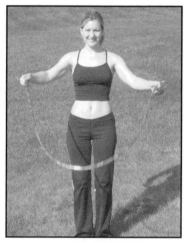

Jump Rope

You can jump rope with or without the rope. You can vary your style by moving forward with skipping, hopping, criss-crossing the feet, boxer's style (alternating heel presses into the floor in front of the body), or twirling the rope backward.

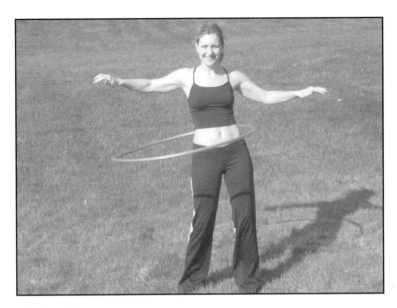

Hula Hoop

You can hula with or without a hula hoop. Stand tall and circle the hoop around the body, or just swivel the hips, to the right for half of your station time. Then, reverse direction and circle to the left for the remainder.

Ball Bouncing

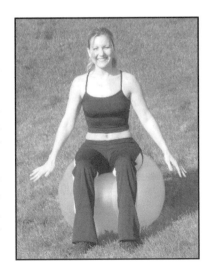

Keep your feet on the floor in front of you. Begin bouncing up and down, keeping bottom in contact with the ball. Your feet can come up off the floor for more intensity. Try moving the arms in various ways to elevate the heart rate, such as small bicep curls, overhead presses or circles to the sides. Sit tall on a stability ball.

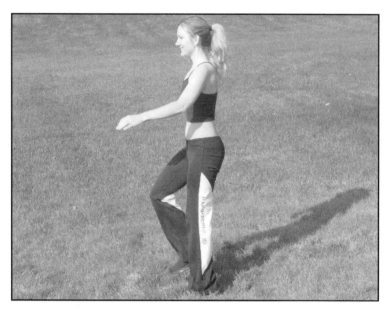

Skipping

Begin standing with your right foot in front of your left. Hop twice in place. On the second hop, quickly switch your left foot to the front, moving forward. Hop twice in place. On the second hop, quickly switch your right foot back to the front, moving forward. Continue alternating and moving around the room.

Some Final Thoughts on CV Exercise

- A perfect body doesn't mean anything if it houses an imperfect heart.
- A warm-up helps you burn calories more efficiently and prepares your body for exercise by increasing body temperature, supplying more oxygen to muscles.
- One hour of vigorous exercise burns approximately 500 calories.
- 3500 calories equals one pound.
- If you exercise every day for one hour and burn 500 calories, you will lose one pound a week.

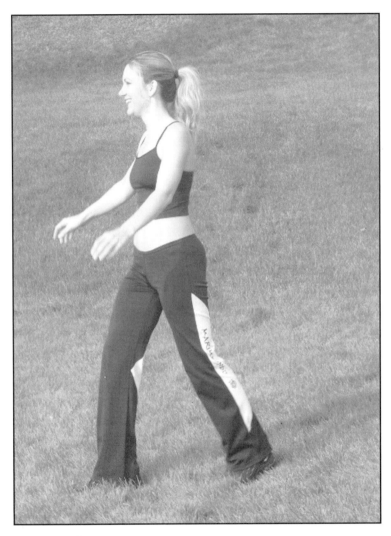

Galloping

Stand tall with your right foot in front of your left. Shuffle-jump around the room, quickly shifting your body's weight between the right and left feet. Halfway through your station time, switch to the left foot in front.

4

Strengthening Exercises

STRENGTH

Improving your strength relies on all the muscles of the body. We use our muscles for everything from holding this book to carrying groceries. One of the superior qualities of muscle tissue is its ability to burn calories 24 hours a day. This correlates to an increase in the body's metabolism.

What this means is that muscle tissue is burning calories for us while we're driving, reading, watching television and sleeping. It helps to burn off the food we eat, keeping it from being stored as fat. The CV system burns off fat we've already stored. This circuit training workout combines CV exercises and strengthening exercises for an effective workout to burn fat and increase metabolism.

Muscles respond to resistance by increasing muscle fiber size and strength, along with increasing the strength of ligaments and tendons surrounding the muscles.

Adaptation occurs quickly, especially if you've strength trained. Muscles have magnificent memory and want to be strong for us. On the flip side, muscle degeneration occurs quickly without appropriate stimuli, causing a decrease in metabolism. That's a motivation to make fitness a way of life. It needs to become a habit and something to look forward to.

Unless we perform regular strength-training exercise, we lose approximately half a pound of muscle every year after age 25. After age 30, muscle mass and strength both begin to decrease. Adding a few strength-training exercises into every week will help prevent the muscle loss that naturally occurs with aging.

The body's strength is dependent on certain factors from gender, age and limb length to the percentage of muscle fibers, point of tendon

While Strength Training, Follow These Basic Guidelines

- Move limbs through a full range of motion, without locking the joints.
- Lift with a controlled speed, using approximately one to two seconds for the lifting motion and three to four seconds for a lowering motion.
- Work slowly and in a controlled manner with each exercise.
- Listen to your body. Take a break when needed.
- Begin gently and gradually work up to a challenging intensity.

insertion and muscle length. It is unrealistic to compare our bodies to with others. Our gains and improvements are as individualized as we are. Be patient with your progress and pay attention to the small gains instead of focusing on a large goal.

Muscles respond to any type of resistance, whether it's a dumbbell, resistance exercise band, full milk jugs, rocks or the body itself. Like the heart and lungs, muscles cannot see, they simply respond to the increased stimuli. Muscles need 48 hours to recover/repair from a workout, so give the body a day of rest between sessions.

The exercises described in this book are safe if the instructions are followed carefully. Please seek the advice of your physician before beginning this or any exercise program. The exercises are divided into muscle groups, largest to smallest. When choosing exercises for your circuit, choose at least one exercise from each muscle group.

Legs

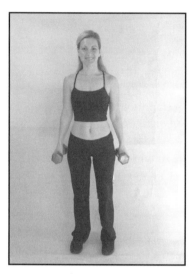 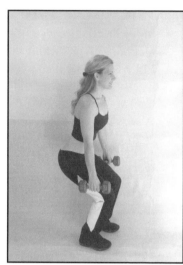

Squats

Stand tall with your feet shoulder distance apart. On an inhale, bend your knees and lower your hips until knees are bent close to 90 degrees. With an exhale, push through the heels, straighten your legs and stand tall. You may use solely the weight of the body, or hold a dumbbell in each hand for added resistance.

Legs

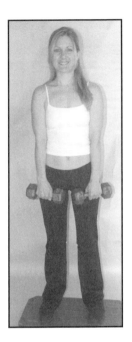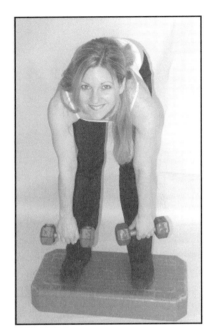

Dead Lifts

Stand tall with feet hip distance apart. Hold a dumbbell in each hand with your palms facing toward your body. Inhale and bend forward from the waist. Keep your spine straight, stomach pulled in and look straight ahead. Only bend forward to a point where you can still look ahead. If the head begins to drop down, pull out of the exercise. On an exhale, squeeze your backside to pull the body back to a standing position.

Legs

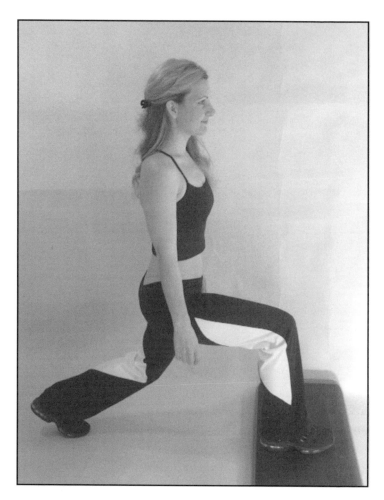

Lunges

Stand facing a bench or stairs. Inhale and step your right foot up onto the bench or stairs. Make sure the full foot comes into contact with the bench. Keep your right knee over the right heel. Bend your left knee slowly lowering the body. Exhale and push off with your right foot to return feet together. Continue alternating legs in a slow and controlled manner. You may add dumbbells for more resistance.

Legs

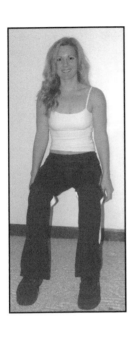

Wall Sits

Stand with your back against a wall. Walk your feet away from the wall, bend your knees and sink your body toward the floor. Keep the knees over the heels and do not bend your knees more than 90 degrees. Press your lower back into the wall and pull the stomach in. The weight of your body presses down into the heels to protect the knees. Maintain this position and breathe!

Single Leg Squat

Stand tall and shift your weight onto your right leg. Bend your right knee slightly and place the heel of your left foot in front of your right foot. Keep the weight of your body on your right heel. Inhale and bend your right knee further, lowering your hips toward the floor. On an exhale, straighten the right leg to the starting position. Spend half of your station time on the right leg, the other half on the left.

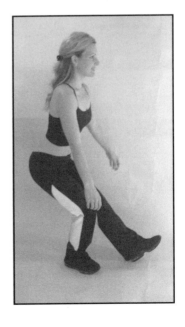

Legs

Wide Leg Squats

Stand with legs wider than shoulder distance apart. Bend your knees and turn the knees and toes slightly out to the sides. Inhale, bend your knees and lower your hips. Keep the weight of the body pressing through the heels. On an exhale, straighten your legs, but keep a slight bend in the knee. You may use the weight of your body or add dumbbells held to the tops of your legs.

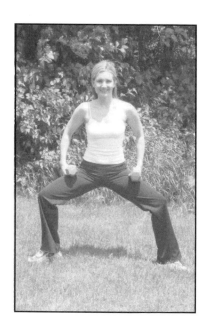

Use Correct Alignment

- Keep the spine straight.
- Pull the stomach in tight, as if trying to squeeze into a tight pair of pants.
- Keep the joints soft, never fully extend or lock a joint.
- Keep knees over the heels, not forward over the toes.
- Keep chin parallel to the floor.
- Keep shoulders over the hips when standing.

Legs

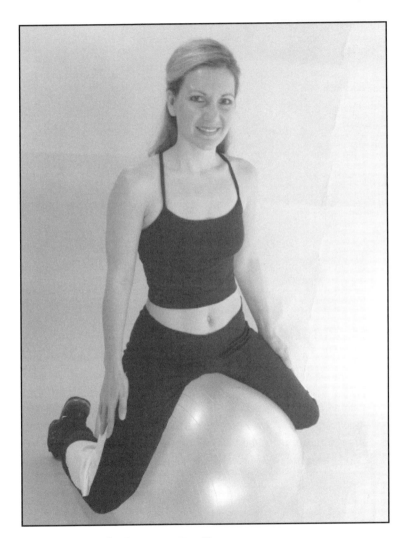

Inner Thigh on Ball

Stand behind your ball and approach it as if you were getting on a horse. Straddle the ball and point your knees toward the floor with feet behind the ball. Using your inner thighs, exhale and squeeze the ball between the knees. Inhale and release the squeeze.

Calves

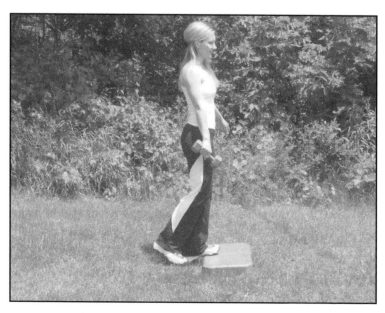

Calf Raises

Place the toes of your right foot onto the edge of a bench or stairs. Allow your left foot to hang off the edge. Hold a dumbbell in your left hand. You may hold onto the wall with your right hand for balance. Exhale and come farther up onto the ball of the right foot, squeezing with the back of the lower leg. Inhale and lower the right heel below the edge of the step. Spend half of your station time on the right leg, followed by the second half on the left leg.

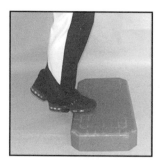 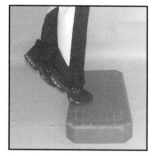

Calves

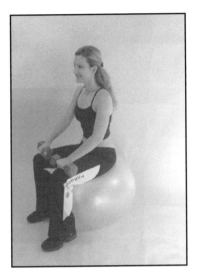 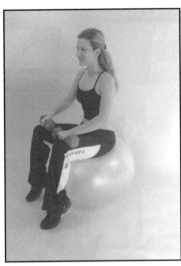

Seated Calf Raises

Sit on your ball or in a chair. Keep your feet on the floor and bend your knees to a 90-degree angle. Hold dumbbells across your thighs and above the knees. Exhale and lift heels, squeezing the backs of the legs. Inhale and lower heels to the floor.

Exercising at Work

You have one muscle in your stomach that is only trained when you pull your stomach in. This muscle aids in posture and in flattening the abdominal area. While at your desk, you can contract and release this muscle by pulling the belly button toward the spine, holding for a count of five and then slowly releasing. Repeat this exercise for as long as possible. It's not one that you have to think about, so doing work at the same time won't be a problem. This is a quick, easy way to strengthen the stomach, improve your posture, and help you look as if you've lost a few pounds!

Chest

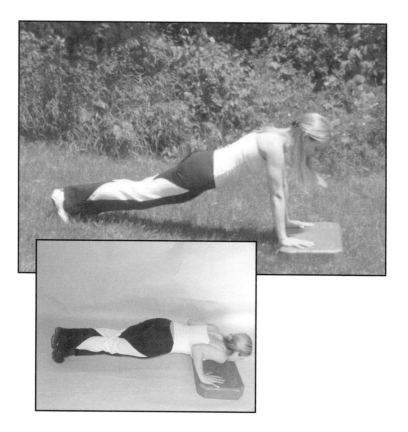

Push-ups

Begin with hands and knees on the floor. Your wrists should be positioned underneath the shoulders. Straighten your spine, tighten your stomach and come up onto your toes. On an inhale, bend the elbows, lowering your chest toward the floor. Keep your focus down toward the floor. On an exhale, straighten your elbows and return to the upper push-up position. For modification, remain on your knees throughout the entire movement. You may also substitute wall push-ups until strength gains are made.

Chest

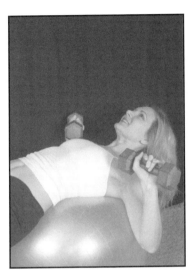 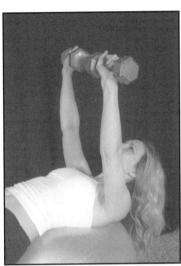

Chest Press

Lie with your back on a ball or a bench. Hold dumbbells in your hands with the arms extended toward the sky and the palms facing towards the feet. Inhale, bend your elbows and slowly lower them to the sides. Keep your hands higher than your elbows. On an exhale, straighten your elbows and press your hands towards the start position. Keep your neck relaxed and the stomach pulled in.

Chest

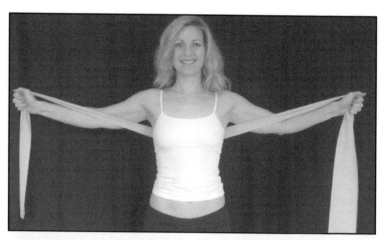

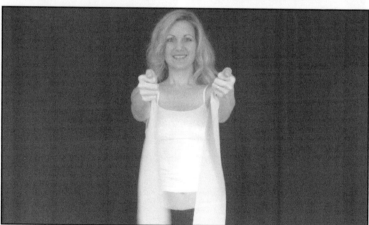

Chest Flies

Stand or sit and wrap an exercise band around your back. Pass the band underneath the arms and take hold of one end of the band in each hand. Begin with your arms extended to the sides. Exhale and close arms together. Concentrate on squeezing the elbows toward each other to feel the contraction in the chest. Inhale, and with control, release the arms back out to the sides. Keep your elbows high and in line with the shoulders and wrists.

Back

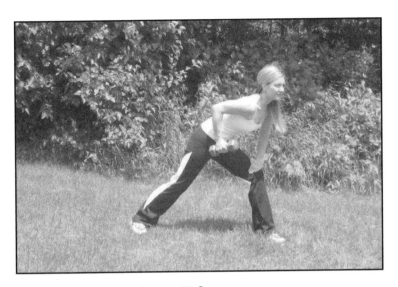

Dumbbell Lat Pull-ins

Stand in a lunge position with your left leg in front of your right. Slightly bend your left knee and place your left hand on your left thigh. Grasp one dumbbell in the right hand and place the right hand next to the left knee with your palm facing toward the knee. Exhale and bring the right hand up toward the right hip. Keep the elbow higher than the body and as close to your body as possible. Inhale and slowly release hand toward the left knee. Spend half of your station time on this side and then switch feet and hands for the other side.

Back

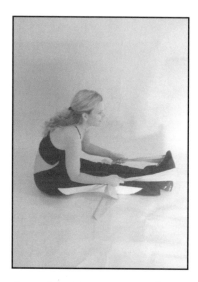
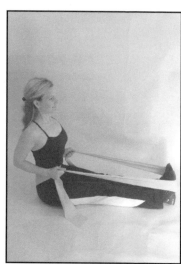

Seated Row with Band

Sit on the floor with your feet placed in the middle of an exercise band. Lean forward from the hips and grasp one side of the band with each hand close to the ankles. Exhale and sit up tall. Pull your elbows behind the body and bring your hands toward your hips. Squeeze your shoulder blades together and feel the contraction in the upper back. Inhale, straighten your arms and release hands toward the ankles.

Lower Back Pain?

- Strong abdominal muscles help to prevent back pain.
- Excess weight across the stomach causes strain in the lower back.
- The back is trying to support the heavy middle.
- Back strengtheners, weight loss and abdominal exercises work together to relieve and prevent back pain.

Back

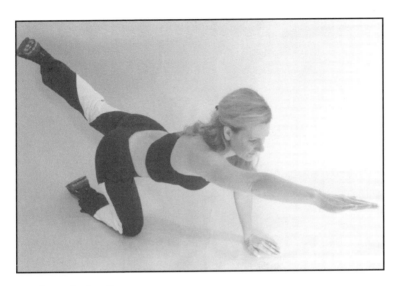

Spinal Balance

Place hands and knees on the floor with wrists underneath the shoulders and knees underneath the hips. Inhale and extend the right arm in front of the body and the left leg behind the body. Exhale and lower the arm and leg. Inhale and extend the left arm in front of the body and the right leg behind the body. Exhale and lower the arm and leg. Continue to alternate sides while reaching out through the fingers and toes to lengthen the spine. Keep your focus toward the floor, allowing your neck to relax.

Abdominals

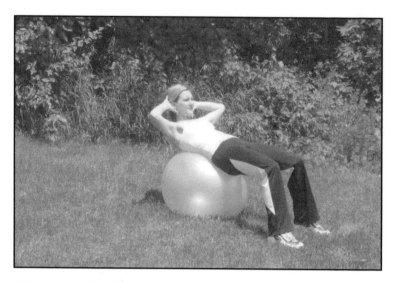

Abs on Ball

Begin sitting on top of a ball. Slowly walk your feet away from you until the ball is behind your lower back. Keep the knees wide to provide stability. Bring your hands behind your head. Keep your fingers open and the thumbs behind your ears. Lay backward over the ball, dropping your head toward the floor. Exhale and use the stomach to lift your shoulder blades off the ball. Keep your elbows wide and look up toward the sky. Inhale and slowly release back over the ball.

Abdominals

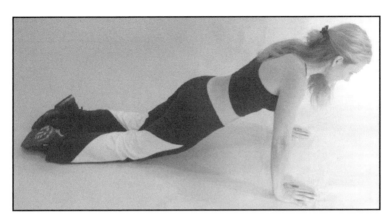

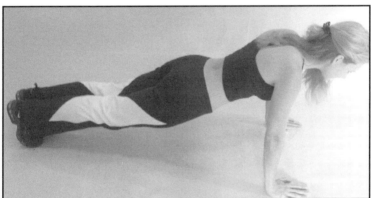

Planks

Place your hands and knees on the floor with your wrists underneath your shoulders. Sink your hips toward the floor and contract the abdominal muscles. For beginners, remain on your knees. For intermediate, come up onto your toes. For an advanced variation, lift one foot off the floor at a time. Keep your focus toward the floor and maintain breathing.

Abdominals

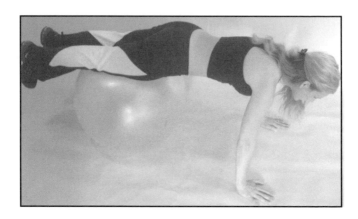

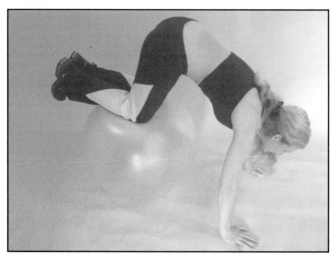

Jackknives

Kneel on the floor with your ball in front of your legs. Place your hands on the floor on the other side of the ball and walk your hands away as the ball rolls down your body. Leave the ball between the knees and ankles. Keep your spine straight and stomach pulled in tight as you exhale and pull your knees into your chest. On an inhale, straighten the legs as you roll the ball away.

Abdominals

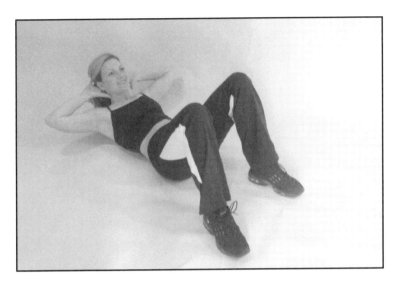

Crunches

Lie on the floor with your knees bent and soles of the feet on the floor. Place your hands behind your head with fingers open and thumbs behind your ears. Tip your hips to press your lower back into the floor. Exhale and lift your shoulder blades off the floor. Keep your elbows out to the side and look toward the sky. Inhale and slowly release the shoulder blades to the floor. Keep your head off the floor until the final repetition.

Getting that "Six Pack"

Simply doing abdominal exercises is not enough to get the "six pack" abs. Many of us have a six pack, but it's covered up by a layer of fat. Cardiovascular exercise to burn off the layer of fat combined with abdominal exercises and a low-fat diet is the only way for that six pack to peek through.

Abdominals

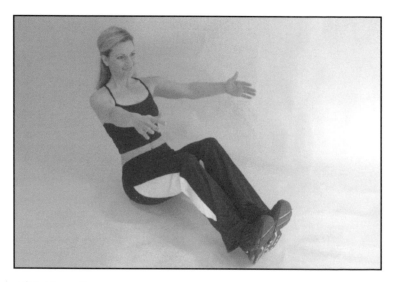

Sit-Backs

Begin seated with your knees bent and toes pointing toward the ceiling. Place your hands on the backs of your legs. Inhale and lower your back toward the floor. This is a very small movement. Keep your spine straight and chest lifted. If you feel your back rounding, you're going back too far. Exhale and return to the seated position. For an intermediate level, extend the arms out at the level of the shoulders. For an advanced level, lift arms all the way overhead.

Abdominals

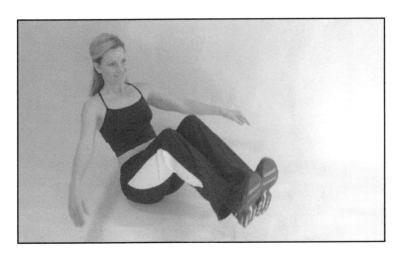

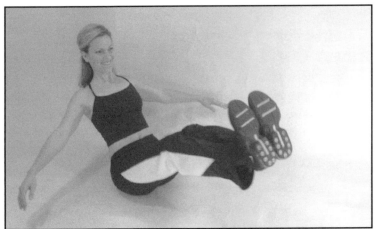

Boat

Begin seated with your knees bent and toes pointing toward the ceiling. Tighten your stomach and find your balance on your seat bones. Inhale and lift your feet off the floor with arms extending to the sides, or resting on the backs of the legs. Hold this position and maintain your breathing. For an advanced exercise, straighten your legs.

Biceps

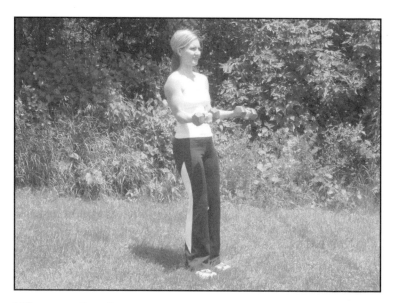

Bicep Curls

Stand or sit with your arms at your sides. Hold a dumbbell in each hand with your palms facing away from your body. Exhale and raise palms toward the shoulders keeping your elbows against your rib cage. Inhale and slowly lower your palms. To perform with an exercise band, place both feet in the middle of the band. Hold onto an end with each hand and bring the hands toward the shoulders, then release.

Biceps

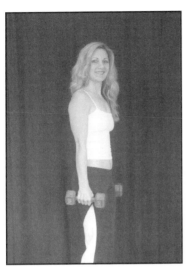 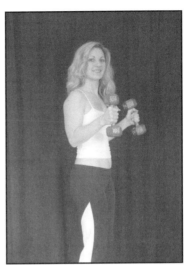

Hammer Curls

Stand tall with a dumbbell in each hand. Begin with your arms at your sides and the palms facing your body. Exhale and lift hands toward the shoulders. Inhale and slowly lower hands to the sides.

Arm Definition: Biceps

- The word BICEPS means a muscle that has two heads.
- We need to train both heads of this muscle.
- The way we do this is to change the hand position.
- The biceps should be trained with one exercise that has the palms facing up and one that has the palms facing down.
- This will activate the most muscle fibers in the front of the upper arms, leading to a more defined look.

Biceps

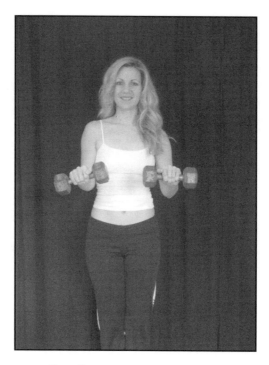

Reverse Curls

Stand tall with a dumbbell in each hand. Begin with your arms straight down and palms facing your body. Exhale and lift the hands toward the shoulders keeping the palms facing the floor. Inhale and slowly lower the hands.

Triceps

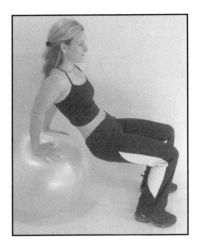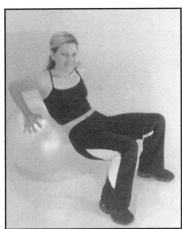

Dips

Sit on a chair, bench or ball and place hands next to the hips with your palms facing down. Walk your feet away from your body, allowing your hips to move away from the base. Inhale, bend your elbows behind your body, and lower your hips toward the floor. Exhale and straighten your arms, lifting your body away from the floor.

Arm Definition: Triceps

- The word TRICEPS means a muscle that has three heads.
- We need to train all the heads of this muscle.
- The way we do this is to change the hand position.
- The triceps should be trained with one exercise that places the palms up, one that places the palms down and one that places the palms toward each other.
- This will activate the most muscle fibers in the back of the upper arm, leading to improved definition.

Triceps

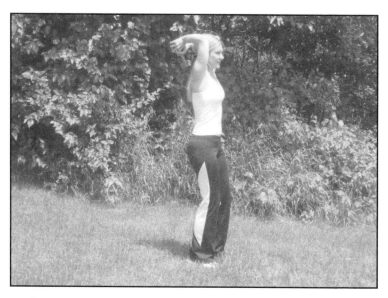

Tricep Extensions

Stand or sit holding a single dumbbell in both hands. Begin with arms straight overhead with the palms facing each other. Keep your elbows as close to your head as possible to provide the best contraction. Inhale and bend your elbows, lowering the weight behind your head. Exhale and straighten arms overhead, pressing the weight up.

Triceps

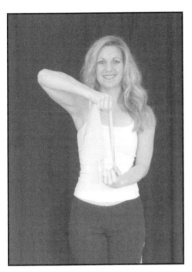 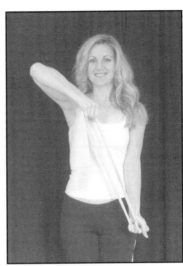

Tricep Band Pull-down

Hold or tie your exercise band into a small circle. Standing or seated, grasp the top of the circle with your right hand. Keep your palm facing the floor. With your left hand, grasp the bottom of the circle with your palm up. Begin with your left arm bent at a 90-degree angle. Exhale and straighten your left arm, bringing your hand toward the side of your body. Inhale, slowly bend the left arm and release to the starting position. Right elbow remains high to support the band. Spend half of your station time on the left arm and half on your right.

Shoulders

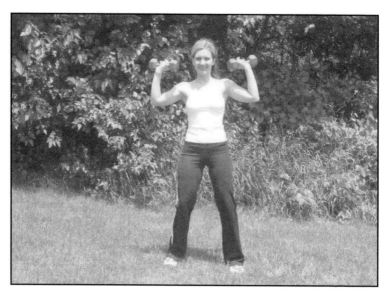

Shoulder Press

Stand or sit with a dumbbell in each hand. Bring your hands up next to your shoulders with your palms facing away and your elbows pointing down. Exhale and straighten your arms toward the sky. Keep a slight bend in your elbows. Inhale, bend the elbows and lower the hands toward the shoulders.

Shoulders

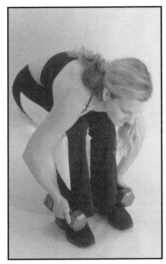 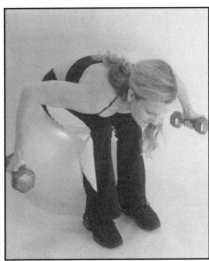

Rear Delt Lift

Sit with a dumbbell in each hand. Fold forward from your waist, bringing your chest toward your legs. Place your hands next to your ankles with your palms facing each other. Bend your elbows slightly and imagine holding a large barrel between your arms. Keeping this arm position, exhale and press elbows toward the sky. Inhale and release hands to the ankles.

Shoulders

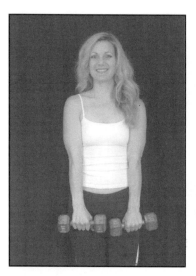 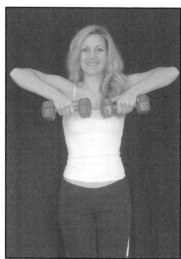

Upright Row

Stand tall with a dumbbell in each hand. Begin with arms in front of your body and palms facing it. Keep your wrists straight and exhale lifting your elbows higher than the shoulders. The weight should remain close to the body and should not come up higher than the chest. Inhale while straightening the arms and lowering hands to the start position.

5

Stretching Exercises

FLEXIBILITY

Flexibility is the joint's ability to move through a full range of motion. As with muscular composition, a number of factors can inhibit mobility, such as genetics, structure, activity level or injury. Improper strength training can lead to muscular imbalances that pull on the bones and shorten muscle fibers. Stretching counteracts these limiting factors and helps to balance muscle groups.

To receive the most benefits from stretching, you should do it every day. After the muscles are warm from the circuit training workout, stretching will facilitate muscular relaxation, tissue waste removal, the return of muscles to normal resting length and improve circulation.

Frequent stretching repairs muscular imbalances from sports or other daily activities. A low-intensity, long-duration (15-30 second) stretch is favored to alleviate joint stiffness and muscular pain. The stretches are static, meaning without movement. There is no bouncing in a stretch.

Stretching, very basically, involves overcoming resistance in a joint by applying force. Elongating the muscle fibers and connective tissue is the goal. Flexibility is specific to each joint, muscle group and individual. The range of motion can also be determined by time of day. You may find you can sink deeper into a stretch in the evening after the body has been moving around throughout the day.

The body should be warm before stretching. Muscles are likened to a piece of plastic. If plastic is bent while cold, it will snap, but if warmed up first, it will gently bend. Muscles react in the same manner. Stretching a cold muscle could result in a muscular pull. A warm muscle stretches deeper and provides relief, not pain.

On the other hand, over-stretching can lead to instability at the joints. To decrease this vulnerability, a combination of stretching and strengthening exercises is recommended.

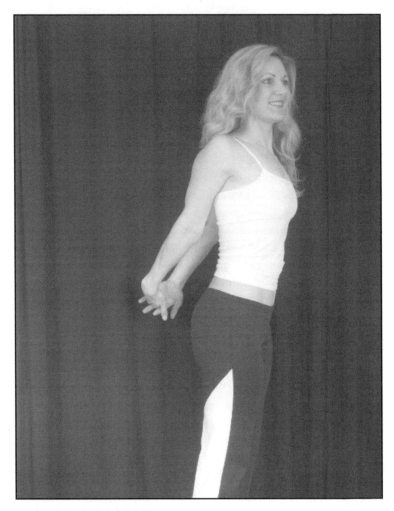

Chest Stretch

Standing tall, lace hands together behind the body. Lift hands with straight arms to a comfortable height. Hold the stretch for a count of 15-20.

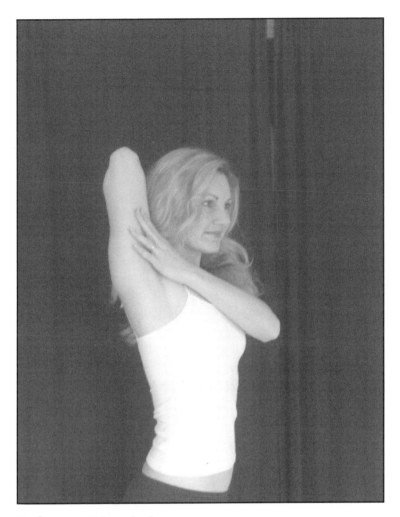

Tricep Stretch

Bring your right arm overhead. Bend the right elbow to bring your right hand between the shoulder blades. The left hand presses on the muscle to assist the stretch. Hold the stretch while counting to 15-20. Repeat on the left arm.

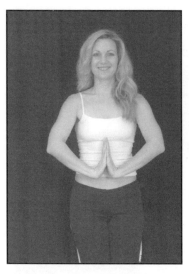 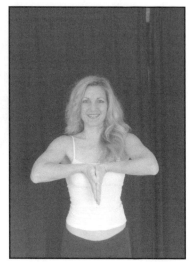

Wrist Stretch

Place palms together in front of the body with fingers pointing toward the sky. Gently lower hands toward the floor, keeping the palms pressed together. Hold for 15-20 seconds. With palms still together, turn hands downward with fingers pointing toward the floor. Gently lift the hands toward the head, pressing the palms together.

Sit at a Computer All Day?

Sitting at a computer or working at a desk causes the body to round forward. This leads to a tight chest and an overstretched upper back. Taking a break three times a day to stretch the chest will conteract this imbalance.

Another result of working on a computer is tight wrists. The above wrist stretch repeated three to four times a day will help alleviate the wrist pain that often accompanies hours of computer work.

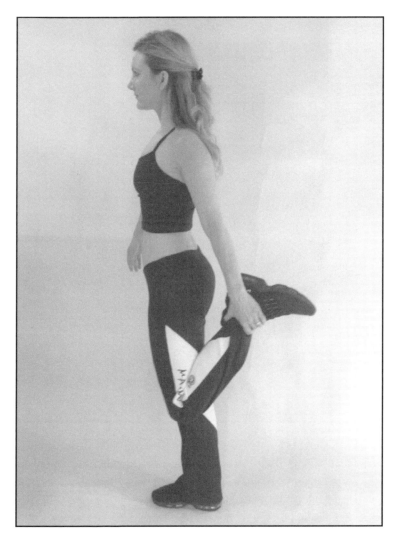

Quadriceps Stretch

Standing tall, shift your weight onto the right leg. Bend the left knee, bringing the left foot toward the back side. Reach back with the left hand to grasp the left ankle. Grasping the toes will pull on the ankle. Keep knee pointing toward the floor. For a more intense stretch, tilt the hips. Hold for 15-20 seconds and repeat on the right leg.

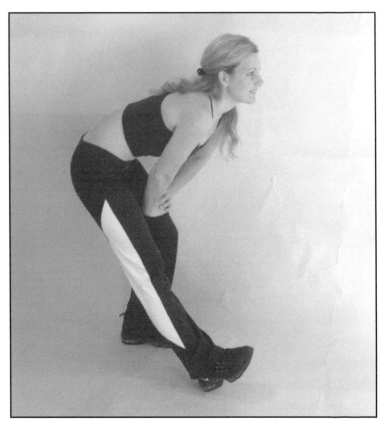

Hamstring

Standing tall, step the right foot out in front of the body. Place the heel on the floor. Both hands are placed on the left leg above the left knee. Bend the left knee, sinking the hips and feeling the stretch in the back of the right leg. Keep your head and chest lifted. Hold for 15-20 seconds and repeat on the left leg.

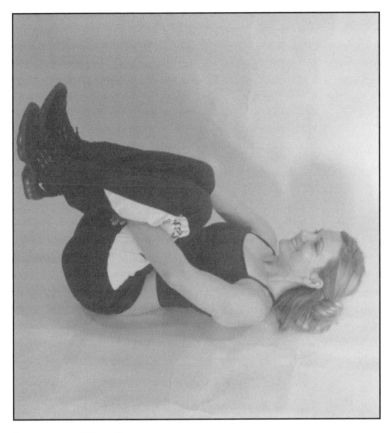

Lower Back

Lie on your back. Bring both knees towards the chest, grasping onto the backs of the legs, behind the knees. Gently rotate the knees in a small circle, and then reverse the direction. Rotate five to ten times each way.

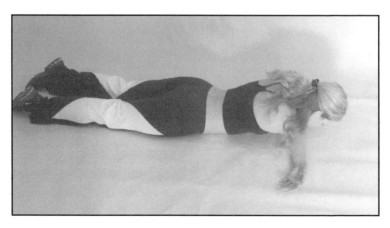

Shoulder

Lie on your stomach with your legs straight. Reach your right hand toward the left side of body at shoulder level with palm facing up. Place the left arm in front of the right, reaching towards right side of the body with palm facing up. Lower head and relax. Hold for 15-20 seconds and then repeat with the right arm in front of left.

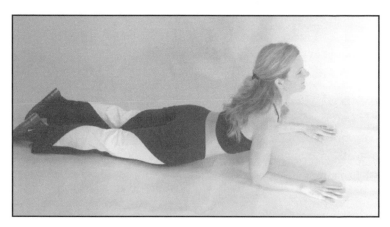

Abdominal

Lie on your stomach. Bend the arms and place elbows underneath the shoulders with palms flat on the floor. Legs are straight. Inhale, lifting your chest away from the floor. Hold and maintain breathing for a count of 15-20.

6

The Circuit Training Workout

The **Basic** Circuit Training workout uses set intervals of 1½ minutes, alternating an aerobic, CV exercise with an anaerobic, or strength training exercise. There is no rest between stations. We move quickly from one station to the next, so it's wise to have the exercises written down, placed in order and have the necessary equipment available.

Begin each circuit with a **Warm-up** — three to four minutes of marching in place, walking around the room, or knee lifts, small lunges, etc.

The following two workouts are included in the back of the book, already written out for your convenience.

For each of the following exercises, see chapters three and four for instructions and perform them in order for 1½ minutes with no rest in between:

Workout 1
Jumping Jacks (page 21)
Wide Leg Squats (page 40)
Jump Rope (page 30)
Push-Ups (page 44)
Jog around room (page 18)
Dumbbell lat pull-ins (page 47)
Front Kicks (page 27)
Abs on Ball (page 50)
Football Run (page 23)
Dips (page 59)
Step-ups (page 19)
Bicep Curls (page 56)
Knee lifts (page 27)

Shoulder Press (page 62)
Hopscotch (page 25)
Calf Raise (page 42)
Cool down: A one- to three-minute walk around the room or slow movements of arms and legs.

Workout 2
Cross Country Ski (page 30)
Lunges (page 38)
Heel Touches (page 28)
Chest Press (page 45)
Football run (page 23)
Spinal Balance (page 49)
Boxer's Shuffle (page 24)
Tricep Extensions (page 60)
Marching in Place (page 20)
Hammer Curls (page 57)
Downhill Ski Jumps (page 26)
Upright Row (page 64)
Ball Bouncing (page 31)
Planks (page 51)
Soccer Kicks (page 29)
Seated Calf Raises (page 44)
Cool down: A one- to three-minute walk around the room or slow movements of arms and legs.
Remember to Stretch!

The **Triple** Circuit Training workout uses a series of three exercises in a repetitive sequence. Two aerobic, CV exercises, then an anaerobic, strength exercise, can be used. Or, two anaerobic then an aerobic can be used. Always warm up for three to four minutes.

Hopscotch (page 25)
Jog (page 18)
Squats (page 36)
Football run (page 23)
Hula Hoop (page 31)
Push-ups (page 44)
Boxer's Shuffle (page 24)
Walking (page 17)
Dumbbell Lat Pull-ins (page 47)
Jumping Jacks (page 21)
Step-ups (page 19)
Dips (page 59)
Downhill Ski Jumps (page 26)
Ball Bouncing (page 31)
Bicep Curls (page 56)
Front Kicks (page 27)
Heel Touches (page 28)
Shoulder Press (page 62)
Jump Rope (page 30)
Cross Country Ski (page 30)
Abs on Ball (page 50)
Cool down and stretch

The **Split** circuit uses alternating periods of work and rest, set at intervals such as 30 seconds of work followed by 30 seconds of rest. The circuit should be shorter and repeated two times. This type of workout is good for the beginner, or when the body's energy level is low. The following is an example:

Jumping Jacks (page 21)
Rest
Wall Sitts (page 39)
Rest
Hopscotch (page 25)
Rest
Chest Flies (page 46)
Rest
Jump Rope (page 30)
Rest
Tricep Band Pull-downs (page 61)
Rest
Jog (page 18)
Rest
Crunches (page 53)
Rest
Galloping (page 33)
Rest
Reverse Curls (page 58)
Repeat entire sequence

The **Roaring** Circuit is based on a set number of repetitions instead of an amount of time. For example, 100 jogs in place followed by 20 squats, 100 marches, and then 20 push-ups. Set your numbers before beginning and stick with them throughout the entire sequence.

The **Repeat** circuit uses the same exercise between the others through the entire workout. This workout is good for the athlete who is seeking sport-specific training. For example:

Push-ups (page 44)
Jog (page 18)
Wall Sits (page 39)
Jog (page 18)
Dumbbell Lat pull-ins (page 47)
Jog (page 18)
Shoulder Press (page 62)
Jog (page 18)
Dips (page 59)
Jog (page 18)
Calf Raises (page 42)
Jog (page 18)
Bicep Curls (page 56)
Jog (page 18)
Abs (page 50)
Jog (page 18)

The **Fartlek** (speed play) training method was developed in Sweden. Unlike traditional circuit training, the Fartlek method uses intervals based upon how you feel. You should maintain one station until your cannot do anymore, and then move on to the next. How you feel determines the length and the speed of each station.

The Fartlek training system may be used when working toward gains in specific abilities. For example, you can run and significantly increase the pace until you can't continue, then pull back and slow down until you recover enough to increase again.

Interval Training is another type of circuit training. Interval training works within the same exercise system, either aerobic or anaerobic.

An aerobic interval training workout uses bouts of exercise designed to increase the heart rate to the 60-80% range, alternating with periods of recovery at low speed and intensity. An example of this would be bicycling at a high resistance, and then at zero resistance. The work and recovery times are the same. If exercising hard for two minutes, recovery is also for two minutes. This should be repeated for 10 times for a total workout of 40 minutes. Higher intensity interval training should be performed by athletes looking to improve their speed and endurance.

An anaerobic interval training workout is designed to increase speed and power. This should be reserved for seasoned exercisers and not for beginners. This type of training carries with it the greatest risk of injuries.

An aerobic workout involves going from one strengthening exercise to the next without rest in between. The amount of weight is set high at intensities of 85-100% of maximum weight. The athlete should include a significant warm-up prior to this workout.

Taking it to the Gym

Circuit training can also be used at your health club. It takes creativity and dedication on your part not to get distracted by the social aspect of the club, and to overcome hindrances such as the distance between machines.

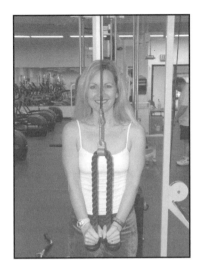

Begin with a warm-up on a treadmill, bike, etc. Choose a weight machine and begin your workout for 1½ minutes. After the strength machine, work your way back to the cardio area and walk, ride or step for 1½ minutes. Continue this sequence until you've strengthened all the muscle groups of the body.

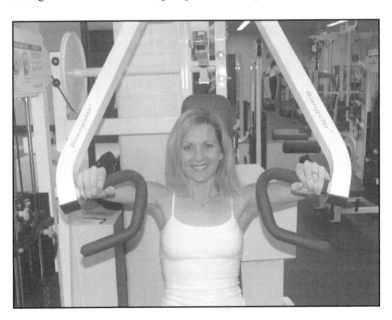

Taking it to the Pool

Another variation on the circuit workout is to take it into the water. Water exercise has the ability to reduce the "weight" of a person by approximately 90%. This results in less stress on our joints, bones and muscles. It provides an adequate workout without the risk of injury or muscular soreness.

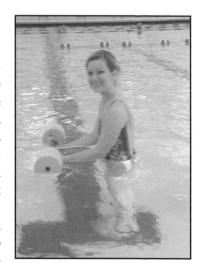

Water exercise provides an alternative to land for those who need a gentle approach. For example, anyone with arthritis will embrace the water for its therapeutic aspects. Those recovering from injuries will also find relief in the water.

Aerobic workouts in the pool are effective for strengthening the heart and lungs. The only difference is in the measure of the heart rate. The water causes the heart rate to be reduced by seven to 15 beats per minute when compared to our land workouts. Therefore, it is important to pay attention to how you feel when doing water exercise instead of focusing on the heart rate range.

The water resistance alone adds strength training. We resist the water 360 degrees around the body no matter which way we're moving. This causes all of the muscles of the body to respond. They fight to keep us upright and stable. With the addition of hand-held paddles or dumbbells we are able to increase the resistance workout.

Many aquatic centers have circuit training classes, so that would be the place to start. If that is not available, setting up a water circuit is simple. The same movements we're using on land can be taken to the water; jog, march, jumping jacks, cross-country ski, skips, etc. For the resistance, exercise bands and water dumbbells can be brought into the pool and be used to strengthen the muscles.

7

Special Considerations/Modifications, Safety Guidelines and Special Populations

Follow these **special considerations** if you:

- are pregnant: please check with your doctor before beginning this or any exercise program. Do not lie on your back for abdominals or other strengthening exercises.
- have hypertension or high blood pressure: please check with your doctor. Avoid holding your breath and holding the dumbbells tightly.
- have shoulder injuries or dislocations: avoid overhead lifting with the weight and use a lighter weight amount.
- have lower back injuries: keep knees slightly bent throughout the workout and avoid dead lifts.
- have upper back injuries: do not drop the head back, keep focus forward, and use caution with overhead lifting.
- have wrist pain, carpal tunnel syndrome, or arthritis in the hands: rest on the knuckles instead of the palms in the spinal balance, jackknives, planks and push-ups. Keep wrists as straight as possible when working with the dumbbells.
- are fatigued: listen to your body and adjust your workout for the day. Use the way you feel to time the stations instead of adhering to a set period of time.
- have knee or ankle injuries: be sure to use stable shoes, and follow your doctor's advice.
- have asthma: always carry your inhaler with you and if you have an attack during exercise, stop.
- have diabetes: seek the advice of your doctor, and have a snack on hand.

Safety Guidelines

- Wear comfortable supportive shoes. This will provide a stable base for all of the exercises to move from.
- Have water on hand and keep well hydrated throughout the workout.
- Set up stations prior to the workout to avoid confusion and to save time.
- Use low-impact alternatives, such as marching instead of jogging, if feeling fatigued.
- Choose a weight that is comfortable to lift for the duration of the station. Do not lift too heavy a weight which could increase risk of injury.
- Keep joints soft, not locked throughout the exercises.
- Breathe throughout all movements.
- Keep the spine lengthened and the abdominal muscles pulled in tightly to protect the spine.
- Wear comfortable clothing that will not interfere with the movements.
- Take a break when needed.
- Only participate in the workout three to four days per week and allow for a day of rest in between.

Special Populations

Circuit training has been proven an effective workout for diabetics. Type 2 diabetics participating in circuit training workouts have shown improvements in functional capacity, lean body mass, strength and glycemic control according to a study published in *Diabetes Research and Clinical Practice* in May 2002. Sixteen subjects with Type 2 diabetes participated in an eight-week circuit training program. Post-exercise blood pressure was significantly lower as were submaximal heart rates. This is good news for diabetics with increased risk for heart disease.

For adolescents with insulin-dependent diabetes, circuit training has been found to be a safe exercise program for improving cardiorespiratory endurance, muscle strength, lipid profile and glucose regulation. *The Archives of Physical Medicine and Rehabilitation* in June 1998 studied the effects of circuit training on 10 adolescent male insulin-dependent diabetics. The group mixed endurance and strength activities three times weekly for 12 weeks. The participants improved endurance and strength while increasing their lean body mass.

For obese adolescents, circuit training has improved functional capacity, muscular strength, and body composition. The study presented in the *Journal of the American College of Cardiology*, May 2004, examined the effect of circuit training on 19 obese adolescents.

A short program of task-specific strengthening exercises and training for children with cerebral palsy, run as a group circuit class, resulted in improved strength and functional performance that was maintained over time, according to *Clinical Rehabilitation* magazine in February 2003.

The *International Journal of Eating Disorders* in July 2001, revealed the results of its study on circuit weight training and the effect on body images of college students. They found that after a six-week exercise program, the 39 participants had a significantly improved evaluation of their appearance, greater body satisfaction, reduced social physique anxiety, and enhanced physical self-efficacy.

Circuit training is a tool that everyone can benefit from. From the older adult to the adolescent, this exercise program results in improved health and fitness, body image, blood sugar and cholesterol levels.

8

Purchasing Equipment and More Information

Selecting proper equipment and footwear is essential to an effective workout program. "Try before you buy" is a good rule to follow. Purchasing equipment is an investment in your health and wellness. Take your time, research your options and make an informed decision.

FOOTWEAR

Shoes come in a variety of colors and sport-specific styles. A good quality shoe from a reputable manufacturer, such as Reebok, Nike, New Balance or Adidas may cost more than a discount store brand, but will last longer and protect your joints from injuries. Poorly designed footwear can lead to discomfort or injury and make participation in exercise an unpleasant experience.

Shoes are important for cardiovascular and other impact exercises. They help keep the ankles stable and the knees and hips in alignment. They also absorb impact between the foot and ground, providing a buffer for shock.

Shoes provide a stable base of support when strength training. Shoes help to protect against ankle roll-over and maintain correct arch support. Shoes also protect the foot from abrasion and strain from the floor, ground or fitness equipment. Refer to the following guidelines when choosing footwear:

- Visit an athletic-shoe store with qualified personnel. These people are trained to fit the shoe to the individual's foot and fitness needs.
- Try on shoes at the end of the day when foot size is at its maximum. Wear the same socks you will wear during the exercise activity.
- Mimic the movements of the exercises in the stores. Don't

worry about looking silly. Take the time to fit the shoe in the store rather than be in pain later.

- A shoe will fit the first time you wear it. If it doesn't feel comfortable the first time, it won't later.
- Try on both shoes. Sizes can vary between left and right feet.

LARGE FITNESS EQUIPMENT

For large fitness equipment such as treadmills, stationary bikes, stair climbers or strength training systems, ask yourself these questions:

- What are my specific training needs? Determine whether you are purchasing for cardiovascular, strength or multipurpose exercise.
- How much can I afford to spend? As with any large purchase, set a budget that you can afford. Stick to that budget to avoid buyer's remorse later.
- How much space can I give to equipment? Envision where you will place the equipment in your home.
- Does the equipment come with the features, warranty, safety and serviceability I'm looking for? Warranty and service can be the deciding factor when choosing between two brands of equipment. If it will take weeks to get parts, or if you have to send the piece to the manufacturer, you might not want that brand.
- Does the equipment comfortably fit my body? This will be something you will be using, hopefully, three days a week. Comfort is a priority. Keep searching until you find the one that fits your body composition.

SMALL FITNESS EQUIPMENT

While the financial investment is not as large when purchasing small fitness equipment, purchasing a quality piece will save having to replace it in the future. It's also a good idea to purchase pieces that will adapt to your changing body. A set of five-pound dumbbells might be sufficient to begin with, but you will get stronger. A set of five-, eight- and 10-pound dumbbells might be the better purchase.

Ask yourself these questions when purchasing dumbbells, stability balls, exercise mats or bands:

- What are my specific needs? Products such as stability balls provide a variety of workouts in one piece of equipment. If strength gain is the goal, a set of progressive resistance dumbbells are needed.
- How much can I afford to spend? The smaller pieces aren't costly individually, but can add up if many pieces are acquired.
- Do I have room to store the equipment? Many pieces of exercise equipment all around the house can become a source of anxiety. Designate a closet or storage area with easy access for your supplies.
- Does the equipment comfortably fit my body? Dumbbells come in a variety of styles, materials and sizes. Test for the perfect fit. Exercise bands come in latex-free varieties for those who have latex allergies. Stability balls come in different sizes depending on a person's height.

For more information on equipment and accessories, or to purchase products:

Fitness Wholesale
www.fitnesswholesale.com   800-396-7337

SPRI
www.spriproducts.com   800-222-7774

Power Systems
www.power-systems.com   800-321-6975

Simple Fitness Solutions
www.simplefitnesssolutions.com   888-283-0292

9

Exercise Adherence and Motivation

MOTIVATION

Motivation is a personal issue. Only you know your reasons for beginning or continuing an exercise program. The following are only motivational suggestions. If one touches your heart, use it. If not, continue seeking until you find your personal motivators.

- Remember the "good" feeling after completing a workout.
- Exercise reduces stress and insomnia, alleviates depression, and aids in weight loss and strength gains.
- Include in the circuits, exercises you enjoy, so you'll look forward to the workout.
- Sign a contract with yourself to exercise three days a week for one month.
- Choose a non-food reward if you fulfill the contract.
- Set appropriate, reachable exercise goals for yourself. It is unreasonable to seek to lose more than one to two pounds per week.
- It only takes a few minutes a day in order to see results. You are worth it! Take that time for yourself.

ADHERENCE

After you begin an exercise program, you may look for excuses to skip some of your workouts. Adherence to a program can be helped along by a few tips:

- Schedule exercise into your day — no matter what.
- Choose the time of day that works for your schedule. Try to make it the same time every day.

- Have all necessary equipment in one place so the workout flows smoothly.
- Keep exercise clothes easily available. If you are working out at a club, keep clothes and shoes in the car.
- Tell family and friends about your decision to exercise. Ask them to ask you questions about your progress. This makes you accountable to others.
- Release any setbacks. Focus on the next exercise session, not a missed one.
- Make exercise a way of life. Consciously choose to use stairs instead of escalators. Park farther away from store entrances. Push-mow the lawn instead of using a riding mower. Walk the dog, etc.
- Talk every day with others who are exercising to help keep your focus.
- Pay attention to the gains being made: better-fitting clothes, increased energy levels, fewer mood swings, etc.
- Evaluate your progress on a monthly basis to make sure you're heading in the direction you've planned for yourself. Make adjustments and changes as needed.
- The best advice I can give to you on fitness is to do a little bit each day. Even when you don't feel up to working out, try to do 10 minutes. Research has found that 10 minutes of exercise three times a day is as effective as 30 minutes all at one time. So put away the "I just don't have time" excuse.

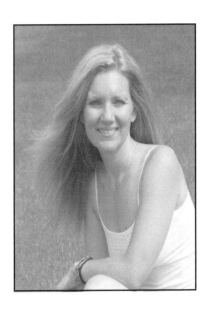

Final Words

If you currently exercise, try incorporating this circuit training into your workout rotations. I hope it provides you with the increased challenge and variety you're looking for.

If you're a beginner, congratulations on making the first step toward improving your health. Ease yourself into exercise, choosing movements that work for your body. Stick with it and soon it will become a habit that you'll look forward to.

Best of luck with this workout and with all of your future exercise pursuits. If you have any questions, I am always available through my website, www.yogaband.com.

Stay healthy,
Lisa M. Wolfe

Cut Out Sample Workout

Use the workout examples on pages 73-74 to set up these cut-outs for your first two circuit training workouts. After that, mix up the stations by using the formats for a basic, triple, split, roaring or repeat circuits.

Jumping Jacks

Wide Leg Squats

Jump Rope

Push-ups

Jog

Dumbbell Lat Pull-ins

Front Kicks

Abs on Ball

Football Run

Dips

Step-ups

Bicep Curls

Knee Lifts

Shoulder Press

Hopscotch

Calf Raises

Cross Country Ski

Lunges

Heel Touches

Chest Press

Football Run

Spinal Balance

Boxer's Shuffle

Tricep Extensions

March

Hammer Curls

Downhill Ski

Upright Row

Ball Bouncing

Planks

Soccer Kicks

Seated Calf Raise